PREVENTING AND MANAGING REVERSE HEART DISEASE

A Complete Guide to Cardiovascular Wellness, Heart attack and risk factors, scientifically proven healing methods, Tips and Techniques

Brandon Oliver

Brandon Oliver

TABLE OF CONTENTS

INTRODUCTON

A comprehensive examination of strategies to counteract and control heart disease. This book is a practical guide for individuals seeking to understand the complexities of cardiovascular health, offering actionable advice grounded in scientific research. Through a clear and accessible approach, it empowers readers with the knowledge needed to make informed decisions about their heart health. From lifestyle modifications to medical interventions, each chapter presents evidence-based insights and practical tips for preventing and managing heart disease effectively. Whether you are seeking to enhance your current health regimen or are dealing with specific heart-related issues, this book serves as a valuable resource to support your healing and discovering process toward a healthier heart and a better quality of life.

CHAPTER 1

What is Heart Disease?

Heart disease, also known as cardiovascular disease, encompasses a broad spectrum of heart-related issues. It stands as the primary cause of mortality in the United States, yet there exist strategies for both prevention and management across various heart conditions. Specifically, coronary heart disease, characterized by inadequate delivery of oxygen-rich blood to the heart due to arterial issues, is prevalent. This condition, alternatively termed coronary artery disease or ischemic heart disease, affects a significant portion of the U.S. adult population, with approximately 20.5 million individuals afflicted, as reported by the Centers for Disease Control and Prevention. While coronary artery disease primarily impacts the larger coronary arteries situated on the heart's surface, another variant known as coronary micro-vascular disease targets the smaller arteries within the heart muscle.

Understanding the Causes and Risk Factors of Heart Disease

The factors contributing to heart disease vary depending on its specific type.

Atherosclerotic Disease

Atherosclerosis, characterized by the accumulation and hardening of plaque within arteries, leads to conditions like coronary artery disease, peripheral artery disease, and carotid artery disease. While the precise cause of atherosclerosis remains unclear, certain factors can initiate artery damage, facilitating plaque formation at the site of injury.

These detrimental factors encompass:

• Smoking

• Elevated blood pressure

• High levels of blood fats and cholesterol

• Increased blood sugar levels due to diabetes or insulin resistance

Plaque consists of fats, cholesterol, calcium, and other substances. Rupture of these plaques can result in blood clot formation, further narrowing the arteries and predisposing individuals to complications like angina, heart attack, stroke, and transient ischemic attacks (TIAs).

Cardiac Arrhythmias

Cardiac arrhythmias denote abnormal heart rhythms, encompassing rates that are too fast, too slow, or irregular. Common triggers for arrhythmias include:

• Congenital heart defects

• Coronary artery disease (a form of atherosclerotic disease)

- Elevated blood pressure

- Diabetes

- Heart valve issues

- Certain medications, including both over-the-counter and prescription drugs

- Smoking

- Excessive consumption of alcohol, caffeine, or drugs

- Stress

Heart Valve Disease

Heart valve disease can stem from various causes. While infectious endocarditis or rheumatic heart disease can contribute to its development, valvular heart disease more commonly arises from heart dilation (or cardiac remodeling), calcium deposits on the valves associated with aging, and congenital cardiac anomalies.

Any of the four heart valves can experience either stenosis or regurgitation. The most prevalent congenital heart valve issue is a bicuspid aortic valve. Among adults, significant heart valve diseases such as aortic stenosis, aortic regurgitation, mitral stenosis, and mitral regurgitation are frequently diagnosed. Although mitral valve prolapse (MVP) is the most commonly diagnosed heart valve problem in adults, the majority of cases are mild and unlikely to cause significant heart issues.

Heart Infections

Heart infections are typically caused by bacteria, viruses, parasites, or chemicals infiltrating the heart muscle. This can occur when microbes from the oral cavity or elsewhere in the body enter the bloodstream and adhere to damaged areas of the heart. Infections may also result from microbes entering the body through skin breaks from surgeries or drug use. These infections commonly affect areas such as the chambers and valves (endocarditis), the pericardial sac (pericarditis), and the myocardial layer (myocarditis) of the heart.

Heart Failure

The primary cause of heart failure is often cardiomyopathy, a condition characterized by abnormalities in the heart muscle. Dilated cardiomyopathy, marked by significant enlargement, thinning, and stretching of the left ventricle, is the most prevalent form. Although the exact cause of dilated cardiomyopathy remains unclear, it may be attributed to heart damage leading to reduced blood flow. This condition can be congenital or result from factors like drug use, heart infections, alcohol use disorder, heart attacks, or other heart diseases such as hypertension and arrhythmias.

Hypertrophic cardiomyopathy typically arises from a genetic heart disorder that induces thickening (hypertrophy) of the heart muscle. It can manifest various cardiac issues, including heart failure. The severity of hypertrophic cardiomyopathy varies widely among individuals and is influenced by specific genetic variants. Additionally, this type of cardiomyopathy can develop over time due to conditions like hypertension or aging.

Restrictive Cardiomyopathy, characterized by the stiffening and rigidity of the heart, is the least common type. It may occur spontaneously or be triggered by conditions such as connective tissue disorders, excessive accumulation of iron or protein in the body, and certain cancer treatments.

Several other conditions can weaken the heart and lead to heart failure:

• Coronary artery disease

• Heart attack

• Hypertension

• Damaged heart valves

• Myocarditis (heart infection)

• Congenital heart defects

• Heart arrhythmias

• Chronic illnesses like diabetes, thyroid disorders, and HIV

• Excessive levels of iron or protein in the body

Acute (sudden) heart failure can be caused by:

• Viral infections targeting the heart

• Allergic reactions

• Pulmonary blood clots

• Severe infections

- Certain medications

- Systemic illnesses affecting the entire body

Genetics also play a significant role in various inherited heart diseases and conditions, including:

Arrhythmogenic right ventricular

Cardiomyopathy: This rare inherited disorder leads to the replacement of heart muscle tissue with fatty, scar tissue, increasing the risk of arrhythmias, heart failure, and sudden cardiac death, particularly in young individuals.

Brugada syndrome: An inherited cardiac arrhythmia disorder where certain drugs and electrolyte imbalances can trigger dangerous arrhythmias due to defects in the heart's electrical activity channels.

Cardiac amyloidosis: A form of restrictive cardiomyopathy where protein clumps replace normal heart tissue, potentially leading to heart stiffness and rigidity, either inherited or caused by other diseases.

Cardiac myxoma: Inherited heart tumor, causing arrhythmias, blood flow obstruction, and embolisms as tumor cells detach and travel through the bloodstream.

Familial dilated cardiomyopathy: Up to one-third of cases are inherited, resulting from genetic mutations passed down from parents.

Familial valvular heart disease: Congenital valve abnormalities, including bicuspid aortic valve, mitral valve prolapse, pulmonary valve stenosis, and Ebstein anomaly, can be inherited due to gene mutations.

 Hypertrophic cardiomyopathy: Inherited thickening of the heart muscle due to genetic mutations affecting heart muscle proteins.

Long QT syndrome: Abnormality in the heart's electrical system, often inherited, but can also be drug-induced, potentially leading to severe arrhythmias and sudden death.

Loeyz-Dietz syndrome: Genetic disorder causing enlargement of the aorta, leading to aneurysms and tears in the aortic wall, often accompanied by congenital heart defects.

Marfan syndrome: Genetic disorder affecting the aorta similarly to Loeyz-Dietz syndrome but with distinct gene mutations.

Familial hypercholesterolemia: Inherited disorder resulting in high LDL cholesterol levels from birth, significantly increasing the risk of atherosclerosis and premature heart attacks.

CHAPTER 2
Strategies to Prevent Heart Disease

Preventing heart disease is achievable through adopting a heart-conscious lifestyle. Below are strategies to safeguard your heart health.

Heart disease, a significant cause of mortality, is influenced by factors like family history, gender, and age, which cannot be altered. However, numerous steps can be taken to mitigate the risk.

To enhance heart health, consider these eight recommendations:

Quit Smoking and Tobacco Use: Ceasing smoking or the use of smokeless tobacco significantly benefits heart health. Even individuals who do not smoke themselves should steer clear of exposure to secondhand smoke. Tobacco chemicals harm the heart and blood vessels, reducing oxygen levels in the blood and elevating blood pressure and heart rate. The risk of heart disease diminishes shortly after quitting, with substantial benefits observed within a year of cessation.

Embrace Physical Activity: Engaging in 30 to 60 minutes of daily physical activity reduces heart disease risk. Exercise aids weight management and decreases the likelihood of conditions like hypertension, high cholesterol, and type 2 diabetes. Gradually build up to the recommended levels if you've been inactive. Even brief bouts of activity contribute to heart health, including routine tasks like gardening or walking.

Adopt a Heart-Healthy Diet: Consuming a nutritious diet supports heart health, regulating blood pressure, cholesterol, and diabetes risk. A heart-conscious eating plan includes ample vegetables, fruits, legumes, lean meats, fish, low-fat dairy, whole grains, and healthy fats like olive oil and avocado. Minimize intake of high-sodium, sugary, highly processed, saturated fat, and trans fat-laden foods and beverages.

Keeping a Healthy Weight: It's important to make sure you're not carrying too much weight, especially around your belly. Being too heavy can cause problems like high blood pressure, high cholesterol, and diabetes, which can lead to heart issues.

One way to check if you're too heavy is to measure your body mass index (BMI), which looks at how tall you are compared to how much you weigh. If your BMI is 25 or more, it means you might be too heavy and could be at risk for heart problems.

Another way to see if you're at risk is by measuring how big your waist is. If you're a guy and your waist is over 40 inches, or if you're a girl and it's over 35 inches, you might have a higher chance of heart issues.

Even losing a little bit of weight can help a lot. Dropping just a few pounds can lower your chances of having high levels of bad fats in your blood, keep your sugar levels in check, and make it less likely for you to get diabetes. Losing more weight can also bring down your blood pressure and cholesterol levels.

Getting Good Sleep: Getting enough sleep is super important for staying healthy. Not getting enough sleep can make it more likely for you to become overweight, have high blood pressure, or even have a heart attack or diabetes.

Most adults need about seven hours of sleep each night, and kids usually need even more. It's best to try to go to bed and wake up at the same times every day so your body gets used to it. And make sure your room is dark and quiet to help you sleep better.

If you always feel tired, even after sleeping enough, you might want to talk to a doctor. They can check if you have something called sleep apnea, which can make it harder for you to breathe when you're sleeping and increase your chances of having heart problems. They might suggest losing weight if you need to, or using a special machine to help you breathe better at night.

Managing Stress: Feeling stressed out a lot can be tough on your body, especially your heart. Some people deal with stress by eating too much, drinking too much, or smoking, but those things can make things worse.

Instead, it's good to find other ways to relax and feel better. Doing activities like playing outside, doing puzzles, or drawing can help you feel less stressed. You can also try deep breathing, yoga, or meditation to calm your mind and make your body feel more at ease. These things can help you feel better and keep your heart healthy too.

Getting Help When Stress Feels Too Much: When you feel really stressed out, it's a good idea to get help from a doctor. Long-lasting stress can make you feel anxious or sad, and it can even cause problems with your heart. If you think you might be feeling really sad or anxious, it's important to talk to someone who can help.

Keeping Track of Your Health: Your heart needs to stay healthy, but sometimes, you might not know if it's in trouble. Doctors can check your blood pressure and cholesterol levels to see if everything is okay. They usually start checking blood pressure when you're a kid and keep doing it as you grow up. If you have certain things that might make your heart sick, they might need to check more often.

Checking Blood Pressure: Doctors check blood pressure by squeezing a band around your arm. They do this every couple of years to see if your heart is at risk. Sometimes, they might need to check more often if you're older or have other things that could hurt your heart.

Checking Cholesterol: Cholesterol is like tiny parts in your blood that can build up and make your heart sick. Doctors usually start checking this when you're a bit older, around 9 or 10 years old. They do it every few years to keep an eye on things. If you're older or have more risk, they might need to check more often.

Checking for Diabetes: Diabetes is when your blood sugar is too high, and it can hurt your heart. Doctors start checking for this when you're older, usually around 45. But if you might have it earlier, they might check sooner. They keep checking every few years to make sure you're okay.

What Happens if They Find a Problem?

If the doctor finds something wrong, they might give you medicine or tell you to do certain things to help your heart. It's really important to listen to what they say so you can stay healthy.

CHAPTER 3

Stress Management Techniques for Heart Disease Reversal

We all face stress and anxiety at some stage in our lives, often seen as an inevitable aspect of modern living. Stress is acknowledged as a significant factor in various health issues, particularly impacting heart health. Whether stemming from insufficient sleep or emotional distress, stress is prevalent among professionals struggling with pressure or job loss, often inducing a sense of helplessness. While the body instinctively reacts to safeguard itself, persistent stress can detrimentally affect overall health, including heart function.

When stress strikes, the body releases stress hormones, which can elevate blood cholesterol, sugar, and pressure, all common precursors to heart disease. Various studies have linked heightened stress levels with an increased heart disease risk.

Nevertheless, there's optimism. By adopting effective management strategies and lifestyle adjustments, you can mitigate stress and lower the likelihood of heart disease. Regular physical activity, a balanced diet, and mindfulness practices like meditation can play pivotal roles in averting heart disease. Stress management forms a crucial component of heart disease reversal initiatives, emphasizing the need to identify and address stress for optimal heart health and overall well-being.

We'll explore practical techniques for managing stress to aid in heart disease reversal. Let's look into actionable steps for reducing stress and reversing heart disease:

Exercise: Regular physical activity is an effective means of reducing stress and enhancing overall physical and mental well-being. Engaging in exercise prompts the release of endorphins, natural chemicals that alleviate stress and elevate mood. Moreover, exercise aids in alleviating muscle tension and fostering relaxation, further diminishing stress levels. Establishing a consistent exercise routine can significantly lower stress levels and contribute to a happier life. Discover activities that bring you joy, whether it involves gardening or taking leisurely walks in your neighborhood. Prior to commencing an exercise regimen, it's imperative to consult with your physician to ensure its safety and suitability for you.

Laughter: Beyond being a delightful experience, laughter serves as a natural stress-relief method with both mental and physical benefits. When laughter ensues, the body releases endorphins, enhancing mood and reducing stress levels. Additionally, laughter can fortify the immune system by bolstering antibody production. Numerous studies attest to the positive impact of laughter on heart health, as it promotes increased blood flow, mitigates inflammation, and reduces blood pressure. Incorporate humor into daily activities, surround yourself with individuals who bring joy, or indulge in watching comedy shows to tap into the stress-reducing power of laughter.

Mindfulness Practice: While traditionally regarded as a spiritual pursuit, mindfulness meditation has garnered attention for its stress-reducing effects. Regular mindfulness practice cultivates awareness of thoughts and emotions, enabling more effective identification and management of stress triggers.

Deep Breathing Exercises: Deep breathing techniques offer a simple yet potent strategy for stress reduction and relaxation promotion. When feeling stressed or anxious, breathing often becomes shallow and rapid, exacerbating feelings of tension and anxiety. Deep breathing exercises counteract this by slowing down breathing and increasing oxygen intake, eliciting the relaxation response and effectively managing stress and heart disease.

Writing: Expressing emotions, thoughts, and experiences through writing can serve as a powerful tool for stress and heart problem management. Writing provides an outlet for self-expression and facilitates processing and reflection on thoughts and feelings. By translating thoughts onto paper, individuals gain clarity and insight into their emotional landscape, aiding in stress and heart disease management.

Eat balance diet: Ensuring a diet rich in plant-based foods provides a multitude of health benefits, especially in addressing heart disease. Your doctor will offer tailored recommendations for heart-friendly nutrition. Plant-based options offer ample fiber, aiding in blood sugar balance and mood stabilization. Fruits, veggies, and whole grains abound in essential nutrients vital for nurturing mental and cardiovascular well-being.

Fostering a Positive Mindset: Embracing optimism effectively diminishes anxiety and depression, common precursors to heart disease. Approaching life with positivity enables adept navigation of frustration and emotional challenges, mitigating stress's adverse effects. Cultivating a positive outlook fosters hope and serenity, pivotal for stress management and overall wellness.

Prioritizing Restful Sleep: Adequate sleep is crucial for stress management and holistic health. Insufficient sleep disrupts hormonal equilibrium, elevating stress hormone levels and intensifying tension and anxiety. Strive for 7-8 hours of nightly sleep and establish a consistent routine to optimize stress management and well-being.

Stress profoundly impacts health and can contribute to heart disease onset and progression. By incorporating the strategies outlined here into your daily routine, you can alleviate feelings of tension and anxiety. Collaborate with your healthcare provider to craft a personalized stress management plan tailored to your individual needs and circumstances.

CHAPTER 4

Heart-Healthy Diet in Preventing Heart Disease

You may be aware that certain foods can heighten the risk of heart disease. However, initiating changes to your dietary habits, although challenging, can commence with simple actions today. Whether you've adhered to unhealthy eating patterns for years or seek to refine your diet, here are eight tips for promoting heart health. Discover which foods to increase and which to moderate. Soon, you'll be on the path to a heart-friendlier diet.

Portion Control: Regulating portion sizes is as crucial as selecting the right foods. Loading up your plate, opting for seconds, or eating until full can result in excessive calorie intake. Restaurant servings often exceed necessary amounts.

Implement these strategies to manage portion sizes and improve your diet, benefiting both your heart and waistline:

• Go for smaller plates or bowls to monitor portions effectively.

• Prioritize low-calorie, nutrient-dense foods like fruits and vegetables.

• Limit consumption of high-calorie, high-sodium options such as refined, processed, or fast foods.

Additionally, keep track of your servings with these guidelines in mind:

• Serving sizes are specific measurements, typically in cups, ounces, or pieces.

• Recommended servings from each food group may vary based on dietary guidelines.

• Estimating serving sizes is a skill that may require tools like measuring cups or scales initially.

Increase Vegetable and Fruit Consumption: Veggies and fruits give you important vitamins, minerals, and fiber without packing on too many calories. Their consumption is associated with reduced heart disease risk and can aid in curbing intake of high-calorie foods like meat, cheese, and snacks.

Adding more veggies and fruits to what you eat can be easy:

• Keep prepped vegetables handy in the refrigerator for quick, healthy snacks.

• Display fruits in a visible location to encourage regular consumption.

• Go for recipes featuring vegetables or fruits as primary ingredients, such as stir-fries or fruit-infused salads.

Go for Whole Grains: Whole grains are rich in fiber and nutrients crucial for heart health and blood pressure management. Swap refined grain products for whole grains or explore new options like farro, quinoa, or barley. Strive for at least half of your grain intake to be whole grains.

Limiting Unhealthy Fats: Reduce the consumption of saturated and trans fats to mitigate blood cholesterol levels and diminish the risk of coronary artery disease, a prevalent cardiac ailment. Elevated blood cholesterol can instigate the accumulation of plaque in arteries, leading to atherosclerosis and escalating the likelihood of heart attack and stroke. (Note: The 2020-2025 Dietary Guidelines for Americans advocate restricting saturated fat intake to less than 10% of total daily caloric intake.)

Below are straightforward strategies to curtail saturated and trans fats in your diet for improved cardiac well-being:

• Trim fat from meat or opt for lean cuts containing less than 10% fat.

• Employ minimal quantities of butter, margarine, and shortening in culinary preparations.

• Substitute with low-fat alternatives whenever feasible. For example, replace butter with low-sodium salsa or low-fat yogurt atop a baked potato, or choose sliced whole fruit or low-sugar fruit spread on toast instead of margarine.

• Scrutinize labels of cookies, cakes, frostings, crackers, and chips, which may harbor partially hydrogenated oil despite being labeled as reduced fat. Although partially hydrogenated oil is no longer permitted in US foods, they may persist in products from other countries. Look for partially hydrogenated oil in the ingredient list, an indication of partially hydrogenated oil. Despite certain fats being replaced by saturated fats in desserts and snacks, it's prudent to limit their consumption.

• Go for unsaturated fats when incorporating fats into your diet. Monounsaturated fats, present in olive or canola oil, and polyunsaturated fats, found in select fish, avocados, nuts, and seeds, offer viable alternatives. Substituting unsaturated fats for saturated fats may aid in reducing overall blood cholesterol levels, though moderation in fat intake is essential due to their calorific content.

An effortless method to integrate healthy fats and fiber into your diet is by incorporating ground flaxseed. These diminutive seeds boast high fiber and omega-3 fatty acid content, demonstrated to lower unhealthy cholesterol levels in certain individuals. Grind flaxseeds in a coffee grinder or food processor, then incorporate a teaspoon of the ground flaxseed into yogurt, applesauce, or hot cereal.

Go for Low-Fat Protein Sources:

Skinny meats, chicken, fish, low-fat or fat-free milk products, and eggs are good sources of protein. Favor leaner alternatives such as skinless chicken breasts over fried chicken patties and skim milk over whole milk.

Fish emerges as a preferable option to high-fat meats, particularly those abundant in omega-3 fatty acids, which can reduce blood triglyceride levels. Cold-water fish varieties like salmon, mackerel, and herring excel in omega-3 content. Additional sources encompass flaxseed, walnuts, soybeans, and canola oil.

Legumes such as beans, peas, and lentils constitute excellent low-fat protein reservoirs. Being devoid of cholesterol, they serve as ideal meat substitutes. Opting for plant protein over animal protein diminishes fat and cholesterol intake while augmenting fiber consumption.

Managing Sodium Intake: Sodium, a naturally occurring mineral found in foods like celery and milk, is also added to processed foods such as bread and soup by manufacturers. Consuming foods high in added sodium can contribute to hypertension, or high blood pressure, as does the use of table salt, which contains sodium.

Since high blood pressure increases the risk of heart disease, it's important to cut back on salt and sodium for a heart-friendly diet. The American Heart Association suggests these things for grown-ups:

• Consume no more than 2,300 milligrams (mg) of sodium per day, roughly equivalent to a teaspoon of salt.

• It is advisable to aim for a daily sodium intake of ideally no more than 1,500 mg.

While reducing the amount of salt added to food during cooking or at the table is a good initial step, a significant portion of dietary sodium comes from canned or Processed items like soups, baked goods, and frozen meals, which undergo manufacturing or preparation before being sold for consumption. Going for fresh foods and preparing homemade soups and stews can help reduce sodium consumption.

If you prefer the convenience of canned soups and prepared meals, consider purchasing products with reduced sodium or no added salt. Exercise caution with foods labeled as lower in sodium, as they may still contain substantial sodium levels compared to homemade alternatives. Sea salt, despite its popularity, offers similar nutritional content to regular table salt.

Another strategy to decrease sodium intake involves selecting condiments mindfully. Many condiments offer reduced-sodium versions, while salt substitutes can enhance food flavor with less sodium.

Strategic Meal Planning: Craft daily menus utilizing the six aforementioned tips. Emphasize vegetables, fruits, and whole grains while opting for lean proteins and healthy fats, and moderating intake of salty foods. Pay attention to portion sizes and diversify menu selections.

For instance, if grilled salmon is on the menu one evening, consider incorporating a black bean burger the following night. This approach ensures adequate nutrient intake while adding variety to meals and snacks.

Occasional Indulgences: Allow yourself occasional treats without derailing your heart-healthy diet. Enjoying a candy bar or a handful of potato chips in moderation is acceptable, but refrain from letting treats become a justification for deviating from your healthy-eating plan. Occasional overindulgence is balanced out over time by consistent healthy eating habits.

In general, restrict added sugar intake to less than 10% of total daily calories. For instance, if consuming around 2,000 calories per day, limit added sugar intake to 200 calories, equivalent to approximately 50 grams of added sugar. Refrain from offering foods and

beverages containing added sugar to children
under the age of two.

CHAPTER 5

Coronary Artery Disease Diagnosis and Treatment

Coronary artery disease (CAD) is a prevalent heart condition characterized by the struggle of the major blood vessels (coronary arteries) to adequately supply the heart muscle with blood, oxygen, and nutrients. Typically, this deficiency is caused by cholesterol deposits (plaques) and inflammation within the heart arteries.

Signs and symptoms of CAD manifest when the heart fails to receive sufficient oxygen-rich blood. Individuals with CAD may experience chest pain (angina) and shortness of breath due to reduced blood flow to the heart. If blood flow becomes completely blocked, it can lead to a heart attack.

CAD often develops gradually over years, with symptoms potentially going unnoticed until a significant blockage occurs or a heart attack ensues. Adopting a heart-healthy lifestyle can aid in the prevention of CAD.

Also referred to as coronary heart disease, CAD symptoms may initially go unrecognized or only arise during periods of exertion. As the coronary arteries narrow further, symptoms may intensify or become more frequent.

Common signs and symptoms of CAD include:

Angina: Often described as pressure or tightness in the chest, angina may feel like someone is compressing the chest. It typically occurs in the middle or left side of the chest and can be triggered by physical activity or intense emotions. In some cases, particularly in women, angina may present as brief, sharp pain felt in the neck, arm, or back.

Shortness of breath: Individuals with CAD may experience difficulty catching their breath.

Fatigue: Insufficient blood flow to meet the body's demands can result in unusual tiredness.

Heart attack: A complete blockage of a coronary artery leads to a heart attack. Classic symptoms include intense chest pain or pressure, accompanied by shoulder or arm pain, shortness of breath, and sweating. Women may exhibit less typical symptoms, such as neck or jaw pain, nausea, and fatigue. Some heart attacks may occur without noticeable signs or symptoms.

If you suspect you're experiencing a heart attack, it's crucial to seek immediate medical attention. Dial 911 or your local emergency number promptly. If emergency services aren't accessible, have someone transport you to the nearest hospital. Driving yourself should only be considered as a last resort.

Risk Factors and Diagnosis

Various factors increase the likelihood of developing coronary artery disease (CAD), including smoking, high blood pressure, elevated cholesterol levels, diabetes, obesity, or a strong family history of heart disease. If you're deemed at high risk, consulting your healthcare provider is crucial, as you may require tests to assess arterial narrowing and CAD.

Diagnostic Procedures: During the diagnostic process for CAD, your healthcare provider will conduct a thorough examination, inquiring about your medical history and any symptoms you may be experiencing. Blood tests are commonly administered to evaluate overall health.

Diagnostic Tests

Several tests aid in diagnosing or monitoring CAD:

Electrocardiogram (ECG or EKG): This painless and swift test measures the heart's electrical activity, providing insights into its rhythm and any potential heart attacks.

Echocardiogram: Using sound waves, this test generates images of the heart in motion, revealing blood flow patterns and potential weak areas caused by oxygen deprivation or prior heart attacks, indicative of CAD or other conditions.

Exercise Stress Test: If symptoms predominantly occur during physical exertion, you may be asked to engage in treadmill walking or stationary cycling while undergoing an ECG. When combined with an echocardiogram, it's termed a stress echo. Alternatively, medication may be administered to simulate exercise effects in individuals unable to physically exert themselves.

Nuclear Stress Test: Similar to an exercise stress test, this procedure integrates ECG recordings with images, offering insights into blood flow to the heart muscle during rest and exertion. A radioactive tracer administered via IV enhances visualization of heart arteries.

Cardiac CT scan: This imaging technique identifies calcium deposits and blockages within heart arteries. Contrast dye may be administered intravenously to enhance image clarity, termed CT coronary angiogram when dye is utilized.

Cardiac Catheterization and Angiogram: During this procedure, a cardiologist inserts a flexible catheter into a blood vessel, typically the wrist or groin, guiding it to the heart with

X-ray assistance. Injected dye highlights blood vessels, pinpointing any blockages. If necessary, a balloon on the catheter tip may be inflated to open blocked arteries, often followed by stent placement to maintain artery patency.

These diagnostic tools play vital roles in accurately assessing CAD, guiding subsequent treatment decisions aimed at managing the condition effectively.

Surgical Options and Interventions for Heart Disease

Heart Surgery

Not every heart issue calls for surgical intervention. Lifestyle adjustments, medications, or non-invasive procedures can often suffice. For instance, catheter ablation employs energy to create tiny scars in the heart tissue, thwarting irregular electrical signals. Similarly, coronary angioplasty, a minimally invasive technique, involves inserting a stent into a narrowed or obstructed coronary artery to keep it unobstructed. Nevertheless, surgery becomes imperative for conditions like heart failure, coronary artery blockages, faulty heart valves, and abnormalities in major blood vessels.

Varieties of Heart Surgery

Numerous heart surgeries are available, with the National Heart, Lung, and Blood Institute enumerating several common coronary procedures:

Coronary Artery Bypass Grafting (CABG):

In this prevalent surgery, a healthy artery or vein from another part of the body is connected to redirect blood flow past a blocked coronary artery. Often, this procedure targets multiple arteries simultaneously and is commonly known as heart bypass or coronary artery bypass surgery.

Heart Valve Repair or Replacement: Surgeons mend or substitute faulty valves with either artificial or biological alternatives, crafted from animal or human heart tissue. Repairing a narrowed valve can involve inflating a balloon at its tip via a catheter, inserted through a major blood vessel.

Pacemaker or Implantable Cardioverter Defibrillator (ICD) Insertion: While medications typically manage arrhythmia initially, surgical implantation of a pacemaker or ICD might be necessary if drugs prove ineffective. These devices, placed beneath the skin, regulate heart rhythms via electrical impulses or shock delivery in response to irregularities.

Maze Surgery: This procedure involves creating scar tissue in the heart's upper chambers to channel electrical signals along a controlled path, halting the erratic signals responsible for atrial fibrillation, a prevalent serious arrhythmia.

Aneurysm Repair: Weak sections of arteries or heart walls are reinforced with patches or grafts to rectify balloon-like bulges, known as aneurysms, preventing potential rupture.

Heart Surgery Innovations

Heart transplant and the insertion of ventricular assist devices (VADs) or total artificial hearts (TAHs) stand as remarkable feats in modern medicine. The former involves replacing a diseased heart with a healthy one from a deceased donor, while VADs act as mechanical pumps supporting heart function, and TAHs replace the heart's lower chambers.

Emerging as a minimally invasive alternative, trans-catheter structural heart surgery holds promise. Utilizing a catheter navigated to the heart via blood vessels accessible from various points on the body, such as the groin or chest, this method requires only a small incision. Procedures like transcatheter aortic valve implantation, MitraClip placement, and WATCHMAN placement address specific cardiac anomalies.

Looking at the Risks

Although often successful, heart surgeries carry risks, including bleeding, infection, anesthesia reactions, and damage to vital organs like the heart, kidneys, liver, and lungs. Stroke and mortality risks increase, particularly for individuals with pre-existing conditions like diabetes or lung disease.

An Anesthesiologist's Crucial Role

Cardiac anesthesiologists play a pivotal role throughout heart surgery. Before the operation, they educate patients about anesthesia procedures and risks, assess medical histories, and adjust medications accordingly. During surgery, they meticulously monitor patients using specialized catheters, employing techniques like transesophageal echocardiography (TEE) to guide surgeons and evaluate surgical outcomes. TEE aids in diagnosing emergent issues like low blood pressure or respiratory distress.

Managing Post-Operative Care

During surgery involving a heart-lung bypass machine, the anesthesiologist administers heparin to prevent blood clotting. Surgeons may temporarily halt the heart's beating to conduct the procedure, with the anesthesiologist overseeing the process of restarting and re-establishing normal blood circulation afterward. Although the idea may seem daunting, the use of this machine is a well-established practice, with over a million cardiac operations utilizing it annually worldwide as of 2013.

Post-surgery, the anesthesiologist monitors anesthesia recovery and assists in pain management. While not always the same professional from the operating room, they continue to provide care in the intensive care unit if needed.

Addressing Post-Operative Pain

As pain management specialists, cardiac anesthesiologists tailor post-operative pain relief strategies to individual needs. Before surgery, they assess pain tolerance to determine the most effective pain management approach, which may involve adjusting narcotic dosages, exploring non-narcotic medications, or considering nerve blocks. Although major heart surgeries generally don't result in long-term pain, short-term discomfort can be managed using various methods such as nerve blocks, nonsteroidal anti-inflammatory drugs, acetaminophen, ketamine, or lidocaine infusion, with opioids used sparingly.

Recovery Period

Recovery duration varies depending on the surgery type and individual health. Following most heart surgeries, patients typically spend at least a day in the intensive care unit before transitioning to another hospital unit for further recovery. The length of hospitalization and overall recovery time at home is influenced by factors like the specific surgery undergone, pre-surgery health status, and any complications encountered. For instance, complete recovery from a traditional coronary artery bypass might take six to 12 weeks or longer, as outlined by the National Heart, Lung, and Blood Institute.

CHAPTER 6

Resistant Hypertension

Resistant hypertension refers to persistently elevated blood pressure levels, typically above 140/90 mmHg, despite the concurrent use of three or more medications aimed at managing it. While most individuals with this condition can eventually achieve a healthy blood pressure range, achieving this goal often involves a process of trial and error with various medications.

What Defines Resistant Hypertension?

Resistant hypertension is characterized by blood pressure levels that remain elevated (at or above 140/90 mmHg) despite the utilization of three or more blood pressure medications. These medicines usually contain the highest recommended amounts of:

• One diuretic (a water pill).

• One calcium channel blocker.

• Either one ACE inhibitor or one angiotensin II receptor blocker (ARB) medication.

Hypertension, or high blood pressure, poses a significant health risk, increasing the likelihood of cardiovascular diseases such as heart and blood vessel disorders.

Healthcare professionals may consider diagnosing resistant hypertension after six months of unsuccessful treatment. Ongoing clinical research is exploring potential procedures to aid individuals with resistant hypertension in the future.

How Prevalent is Resistant Hypertension?
Approximately 29% of adults in the U.S. have high blood pressure, with around 12% of them falling into the resistant hypertension category.

Symptoms and Causes

What are the symptoms of resistant hypertension?

Many individuals can live for years without being aware they have hypertension. However, untreated high blood pressure poses serious health risks. Although symptoms may not always be noticeable, some people may experience headaches, chest pressure, or shortness of breath.

Regular monitoring of blood pressure is crucial, particularly as individuals age. Home monitoring using a reliable electronic device, readily available at most drugstores or online, can be a convenient tool in managing hypertension.

Understanding the Etiology of Resistant Hypertension

The genesis of resistant hypertension encompasses multifaceted factors ranging from lifestyle choices to pharmaceutical interventions and underlying medical conditions.

Lifestyle and Dietary Factors

• Having a higher body mass index (BMI) than 25.

• Not being active regularly, with little physical activity.

• Consumption of sodium-rich foods.

• Excessive alcohol consumption.

Pharmaceutical Influences: Various medications, both prescription and over-the-counter, can exacerbate blood pressure management difficulties. Examples include nonsteroidal anti-inflammatory drugs (NSAIDs) such as ibuprofen and naproxen, nasal decongestants, oral contraceptives, and certain herbal supplements like ginseng and licorice.

Underlying Medical Conditions: Certain treatable secondary conditions can contribute to resistant hypertension. These include primary hyperaldosteronism, renal artery stenosis, chronic kidney disease (CKD), sleep apnea, pheochromocytoma, aortic narrowing, and Cushing syndrome.

Risk Factors Associated with Resistant Hypertension:

• Presence of chronic kidney disease

• Diabetes

• African American ethnicity

• Male gender assignment at birth.

Complications Arising from Resistant Hypertension:

• Individuals grappling with resistant hypertension face heightened risks of stroke, kidney disease, and heart failure compared to those with well-regulated blood pressure levels.

Diagnostic Approach

• Diagnosis entails meticulous evaluation by healthcare providers to ensure accurate blood pressure readings, adherence to prescribed medications, and exclusion of white coat syndrome.

• Detailed medical history interrogation, physical examination for signs like hypertensive retinopathy, and laboratory investigations including urine and blood tests are integral to the diagnostic process.

• Imaging modalities such as X-rays, ultrasound, and computed tomography scans may be employed to assess adrenal gland and kidney artery integrity, with sleep studies often recommended to investigate potential sleep apnea.

Management Strategies

• Treatment modalities encompass a blend of lifestyle modifications and pharmacological interventions.

• Lifestyle adjustments involve salt and alcohol restriction, substitution of NSAIDs with acetaminophen for pain relief, and adoption of regular aerobic exercise sessions lasting at least 30 minutes daily.

Pharmaceutical Interventions

Efforts to address resistant hypertension often commence with ensuring adherence to medication regimens. Surprisingly, approximately 40% of cases stem from non-adherence to prescribed treatments. Consistency in medication intake, including correct dosages and frequency, is paramount for efficacy.

Should challenges in adhering to medication arise, open dialogue with healthcare providers is imperative. Discussion may revolve around mitigating side effects hindering compliance, potentially necessitating a switch to alternative medications or formulations. Augmenting therapy with additional medications may be necessary if initial treatment proves insufficient, sometimes requiring a combination of four or five antihypertensive agents.

Commonly prescribed classes of antihypertensive medications include diuretics, calcium channel blockers, and ACE inhibitors/angiotensin receptor blockers (ARBs). Adjustments, such as doubling diuretic doses or introducing aldosterone antagonists like spironolactone, may be warranted based on individual potassium levels. Beta-blockers could also be considered in certain cases.

Treatment Side Effects

Despite their efficacy, antihypertensive medications may elicit side effects, including dizziness, headaches, increased urination frequency, constipation, dry cough, and fatigue.

Preventive Measures

Adhering to prescribed medication regimens and implementing lifestyle modifications can mitigate the risk of developing resistant hypertension:

• Compliance with medication instructions.

• Maintenance of a healthy weight.

• Regular exercise totaling 150 minutes weekly, distributed across three to five sessions.

• Reduction of dietary salt intake.

• Moderation of alcohol consumption.

• Ensuring adequate nightly rest.

Prognosis

While most individuals with resistant hypertension can achieve blood pressure control through medication, individualized approaches may be necessary. Adjustments, such as switching to potent diuretics or modifying medication timing, may be explored. Despite management efforts, individuals with resistant hypertension face elevated risks of heart failure, heart attack, stroke, kidney disease, and mortality. Regular monitoring and proactive management strategies are essential for optimizing outcomes.

Caring for yourself when living with high blood pressure involves consistent, daily efforts. Here are key steps:

Medication Adherence: Take your blood pressure medications as prescribed, following the recommended times and dosages.

Dietary Restrictions: Limit your intake of salt and alcohol, as they can raise blood pressure. Avoiding processed foods and restaurant meals, which often contain high levels of salt, can be beneficial.

Regular Checkups: Attend regular checkup appointments with your healthcare provider to monitor your blood pressure and overall health.

Physical Activity: Engage in regular exercise to help manage your blood pressure. Try to do at least 150 minutes of moderate-intensity aerobic exercise each week, splitting it up over a few days.

Healthy Weight: Maintain a weight that is healthy for your body type and height. This can help lower your blood pressure and reduce the risk of other health issues.

Home Blood Pressure Monitoring

Regularly check your blood pressure at home, as instructed by your healthcare provider, to monitor changes and ensure your medications are working effectively.

Foods to Avoid

• Salt-rich foods, including processed foods and restaurant meals.

• Alcohol, which has the potential to increase blood pressure.

When to Seek Medical Attention

1. Medication Issues: If you have difficulty taking your prescribed medications.

2. Persistent High Readings: If your blood pressure remains high despite adhering to your medication regimen.

When to Go to the Emergency Room

In the event of a hypertensive crisis, characterized by a sudden spike in blood pressure (180/120 mmHg) and symptoms such as headaches, chest pounding, dizziness, or shortness of breath.

CHAPTER 7

Heart Attack Recovery and Rehabilitation

Heart attack recovery typically spans from two weeks to three months. During this period, it's crucial to adopt lifestyle adjustments aimed at reducing the risk of future cardiac events. These changes encompass integrating more physical activity into your daily routine, adhering to a heart-healthy diet, and ceasing smoking. Participation in a cardiac rehabilitation program can facilitate the initial steps toward implementing these changes.

What is the typical duration needed for recuperation after experiencing a heart attack?

The recovery duration from a heart attack, medically known as myocardial infarction, varies from two weeks to three months. Once fully recuperated, you can resume your professional responsibilities and daily activities.

Several factors influence the duration of recovery, including the severity of the heart attack, the promptness of treatment, the type of treatment administered (open-heart surgery or percutaneous coronary intervention), your overall health, and any existing medical conditions. Consulting your healthcare provider can provide insights into your specific recovery timeline.

What should I anticipate during heart attack recovery?

Transitioning back home after a heart attack might evoke feelings of apprehension or uncertainty. You might have inquiries regarding the normalcy of your recovery process or feel uneasy about being away from your medical support team. Additionally, loved ones may seek guidance on how to best assist you. As you gradually reintegrate into your regular routine, expect changes in various aspects, including activity level, exercise regimen, dietary habits, emotional well-being, and sexual activity.

Striking a balance between rest and activity is paramount during recovery. Sufficient rest aids in healing, while gradually resuming normal activities is essential for a robust recovery. Regular exercise plays a crucial role, and your healthcare provider will offer guidance in this regard.

Activity Level

During the initial week post-discharge, fatigue or weakness may prevail, owing to the heart muscle damage and the adjustment to increased mobility after a period of bed rest. Gradually easing into daily activities is advisable. Below are some tips for the initial recovery phase:

• Dressing up each morning and attending to personal hygiene tasks.

• Engaging in light household chores like folding laundry, cooking, gardening, dusting, and dishwashing.

• Managing activities by pacing yourself and taking breaks as needed.

• Limiting stair climbing, unless advised otherwise by your provider.

• Avoiding heavy lifting, pushing, or pulling until clearance is received from your provider.

• Adhering to your provider's instructions regarding driving, returning to work, and engaging in more strenuous activities.

• Following additional restrictions, if any, particularly after heart catheterization.

Exercise for Heart Attack Recovery

Exercise is pivotal for recovery, and enrolling in a cardiac rehabilitation program offers a structured and supervised environment for safe physical activity. This program also assists in implementing lifestyle modifications conducive to long-term health, such as dietary improvements, stress management, and tobacco cessation. Discussing available cardiac rehab programs with your healthcare provider is advisable.

After completing cardiac rehab, integrating exercise into your daily routine remains crucial. If you weren't previously active, the idea of regular exercise might seem daunting. However, cardiac rehab can assist you in gradually incorporating more movement into your day. By the end of the program, you'll feel prepared to continue independently. Remember, many others have faced similar challenges, and progress comes from consistent, small steps.

Regarding diet for heart attack recovery, prioritizing a heart-healthy eating plan is vital to prevent future cardiovascular issues. While various options exist, research favors the Mediterranean Diet for its heart-protective benefits. This diet emphasizes:

• Centering meals around plant-based foods such as fruits, vegetables, legumes, and whole grains.

• Incorporating healthy fats from sources like olive oil, avocados, and nuts.

• Consuming moderate amounts of seafood, lean poultry, eggs, and low-fat dairy.

• Restricting intake of red meat, fried foods, and sugary treats.

Experiencing emotions like depression, anger, or fear after a heart attack is common.

However, these feelings typically subside with time as you resume regular activities. Here are strategies to manage these emotions effectively:

• Maintain a daily routine by getting dressed and avoiding excessive time in bed.

• Engage in daily walks, adhering to exercise guidelines provided by your healthcare provider.

• Gradually reintegrate into hobbies and social interactions, while being mindful of pacing yourself.

• Share your emotions with supportive individuals such as friends, family, counselors, or support groups.

• Prioritize adequate sleep to avoid fatigue and irritability, while minimizing excessive daytime napping.

• Participate in a cardiac rehab program, which provides both physical and emotional support.

• Don't hesitate to ask questions or seek clarification from your healthcare team regarding your condition and treatment plan. Empowering yourself with knowledge about cardiovascular health enables informed decision-making to support your well-being.

When considering the resumption of sexual activity after a heart attack, the timing largely depends on the type of treatment received and your overall well-being. For individuals who underwent open-heart surgery, it's essential to allow four to six weeks for the breastbone to heal before engaging in sexual activity.

For those who didn't undergo surgery, sexual activity might be feasible as early as two to four weeks post-heart attack. However, it's crucial to assess your energy levels and physical comfort. If you can climb two flights of stairs without significant fatigue or chest pain, you likely have adequate energy for sexual activity.

As you readjust to your routine, consider the following tips:

• Openly communicate with your partner about your energy levels and feelings.

• Explore alternative ways to share intimacy with your partner.

• Go for sexual activity when you're well-rested and physically at ease.

• Allow at least two hours to pass after consuming a heavy meal before engaging in sexual activity.

• Talk to your doctor if you have any worries or questions. Heart disease and certain medications can contribute to sexual dysfunction, and seeking support is essential.

Regarding the recovery of the heart after a heart attack, while the heart can indeed recuperate, it's a gradual process. The heart attack typically leaves behind scar tissue, which may result in some permanent damage. Several factors influence the extent of this damage:

• Timeliness of treatment: Swift treatment minimizes heart damage.

• Location of the blockage: The affected coronary artery dictates the extent of damage, as it supplies blood to specific areas of the heart muscle.

The heart muscle typically requires around two months to heal, but residual scar tissue can compromise its pumping ability over time. This can eventually lead to complications like heart failure. It's essential to discuss the extent of heart damage and long-term expectations with your healthcare provider.

Can you achieve a complete recovery from a heart attack? Many individuals do fully recover and go on to lead long, healthy lives post-heart attack. Yet, it's important to pay attention to the potential dangers involved. Approximately 1 in 5 individuals aged 45 or older experience a second heart attack within five years, underscoring the importance of preventive measures in reducing your risk and ensuring long-term wellness.

Preventing a recurrence

Following a heart attack, prioritizing actions to prevent further heart damage is paramount. Your healthcare provider will offer personalized advice tailored to your specific circumstances. Below are some general strategies to maintain heart health:

• Adherence to medication

Your provider will prescribe medications aimed at:

- Preventing future blood clots.
- Reducing the workload on your heart, enhancing its function and aiding in recovery.
- Lowering cholesterol levels.

Sometimes, extra medications might be given to handle:

- Irregular heartbeats (arrhythmias).
- High blood pressure.
- Angina (chest pain or discomfort).
- Heart failure.

It's crucial to understand your medications fully, including their purpose, potential side effects, and dosing schedule. Take all medications as prescribed, even if you feel well. If you experience any side effects, communicate them to your provider promptly. Maintain a list of medications with you at all times, including their names, purposes, dosages, and timing.

• Lifestyle modifications

While certain risk factors for coronary artery disease, such as age or family history, are beyond your control, you can mitigate others. Discuss strategies with your provider to:

Quit smoking, vaping, or using tobacco products, as tobacco use significantly elevates the risk of coronary artery disease.

Moderate or eliminate alcohol consumption based on your provider's recommendations.

Adopt a dietary plan that promotes lower cholesterol levels, such as the Mediterranean Diet or another suitable option identified by your provider or a dietitian.

Maintain a healthy weight, as excess weight strains the heart and increases the risk of hypertension, high cholesterol, and diabetes. Consult your provider to determine your ideal weight and develop a plan to achieve it.

To maintain heart health and reduce the risk of future heart issues, it's important to integrate exercise into your daily routine. A regular exercise program enhances energy levels, lowers cholesterol, manages weight, and reduces stress. Before starting any exercise plan, consult your healthcare provider for guidance.

Proper management of diabetes is also crucial, as research indicates a link between high blood sugar and the progression of coronary artery disease. Dietary modifications, exercise, and medications can help control diabetes effectively.

Additionally, managing high blood pressure is essential, as it can damage the lining of coronary arteries and lead to coronary artery disease. Maintaining a low-sodium diet, engaging in regular exercise, and adhering to prescribed medications can help keep blood pressure within a healthy range.

Incorporating relaxation techniques such as yoga, meditation, or deep breathing exercises into your routine can help manage stress and anger, both of which increase the risk of coronary artery disease.

Regular heart checkups with your healthcare provider are crucial. You'll typically have a follow-up appointment four to six weeks after leaving the hospital to monitor your recovery progress. Your provider may recommend diagnostic tests like exercise stress tests at regular intervals to monitor your heart health and detect any new or worsening blockages.

It's important to promptly contact your healthcare provider if you experience symptoms such as more frequent or intense angina, shortness of breath (especially at rest), dizziness, or irregular heartbeats.

If you experience angina, which indicates your heart isn't receiving sufficient oxygen-rich blood, follow your provider's advice. Stop activity, sit down and rest, and if you have nitroglycerin, take one tablet under your tongue or spray it under your tongue. If chest pain doesn't go away after five minutes, dial 911 or your local emergency number. Do not drive yourself to the hospital; emergency personnel can provide immediate care. Carry your nitroglycerin with you at all times, and replace it every six months if opened.

CHAPTER 8

Revolutionary Approaches in Managing Cardiovascular Disorders

A concise overview of cardiovascular disease

Cardiovascular disease (CVD) encompasses a range of afflictions affecting the heart and blood vessels, including coronary heart disease, irregular heart rhythms, heart failure, and strokes. These conditions often stem from a process known as atherosclerosis, wherein arterial plaque buildup impedes blood flow, potentially leading to severe complications.

The intricacy of CVD lies in its multifaceted nature and its intersection with various risk factors, such as hypertension, diabetes, high cholesterol, smoking, obesity, and a sedentary lifestyle. Gaining a comprehensive understanding of these maladies is paramount, given that they rank as the primary cause of global mortality and morbidity. Consequently, effective prevention, diagnosis, and treatment strategies are imperative.

The global health ramifications of cardiovascular disease

Cardiovascular disease poses a significant public health challenge on a global scale. According to the World Health Organization, it accounts for approximately 17.9 million deaths annually, comprising nearly a third of all global mortality. CVD affects populations across the spectrum of socioeconomic status, albeit with discrepancies in access to care and treatment quality.

The economic toll of CVD is substantial, encompassing not only direct healthcare costs but also productivity losses due to illness and premature death. Addressing this challenge demands concerted international efforts to enhance prevention, early detection, and treatment accessibility, thereby mitigating the societal and individual impacts of these conditions.

Conventional approaches to treating cardiovascular disease

Traditional interventions for CVD primarily aim at symptom management, complication prevention, and risk factor modification. These encompass a blend of pharmaceuticals, such as anti-hypertensive, anticoagulants, and statins, alongside surgical procedures like angioplasty or coronary artery bypass grafting. Additionally, cardiac rehabilitation programs, integrating exercise regimens, educational components, and psychological support, play a pivotal role in patients' recuperation.

While conventional treatments have proven effective, they come with limitations such as side effects, costs, and the need for long-term adherence. Furthermore, they may not always repair existing cardiac damage, which has spurred interest in more innovative and personalized approaches.

Innovations in Cardiovascular Disease Treatment

Gene Therapy for Cardiovascular Disease:

Gene therapy is revolutionizing CVD treatment by correcting or compensating for defective genes responsible for the disease. Progress in developing safe and effective viral and non-viral vectors for gene transfer has been significant. This approach holds promise for targeted treatments capable of regenerating damaged heart tissue and restoring cardiac function.

Clinical trials are assessing gene therapy's efficacy in treating heart failure and angina pectoris. Challenges such as precision, durability, and safety remain, but advancements could transform CVD management.

Advanced Imaging Technologies

Medical imaging is crucial for CVD diagnosis, and advanced techniques are enhancing cardiac disease visualization and assessment. Cardiac MRI, PET, and SPECT provide detailed images, aiding in accurate cardiac structure and function evaluation.

These technologies are essential for planning surgeries, monitoring treatment effectiveness, and advancing research by improving understanding of CVD mechanisms and facilitating new therapy development.

Brandon Oliver

Nanotechnology in Cardiovascular Disease Treatment

Nanotechnology stands at the forefront of innovation in CVD treatment, utilizing nanoparticles to deliver drugs with precision, minimizing side effects and enhancing efficacy. These nanoparticles can be engineered to target diseased cells or tissues directly, delivering medication precisely where needed. Additionally, nanotechnologies show promise in tissue regeneration and bioengineering, with nanomaterials being developed to repair or replace damaged heart tissue, potentially offering alternatives to conventional treatments. While still in its early stages, this approach holds potential to revolutionize cardiac patient care.

Impact and Future Prospects: Innovative approaches like gene therapy, advanced imaging technologies, and nanotechnologies have demonstrated significant enhancements in clinical outcomes. Gene therapy, for instance, targets the root cause of specific heart diseases, presenting a more sustainable solution compared to symptomatic treatments. Advanced imaging technologies improve diagnostic precision and tailor surgical interventions to individual patients, while nanotechnologies offer targeted and minimally invasive drug delivery.

These advancements not only extend patients' lives but also enhance their quality of life by reducing hospitalizations, physical limitations, and psychological burdens associated with CVD. They offer hope to patients previously limited by treatment options.

Challenges in Implementation: Despite their promise, integrating these innovations into clinical practice faces challenges. Regulatory hurdles, high development costs, and specialized healthcare professional training are barriers to widespread adoption. Additionally, equitable access to advanced treatments is a concern, potentially exacerbating health disparities between different populations and regions.

Rigorous evaluation of new therapies' long-term safety and efficacy through extensive clinical trials is imperative, demanding significant time and resources. Nevertheless, continued commitment from researchers, clinicians, and policymakers is crucial for overcoming these challenges and advancing CVD treatment.

Future Directions: The future of CVD treatment appears promising, with ongoing advancements in research and technology. Personalized medicine, tailored to each patient's genetic, environmental, and lifestyle factors, is a focus. Integration of artificial intelligence and big data analysis holds potential to transform CVD prevention, diagnosis, and treatment.

As scientific knowledge expands, expect the emergence of even more targeted and less invasive therapies. International collaboration and robust research funding are essential for realizing these innovations' potential and ensuring equitable access to benefits worldwide, irrespective of geography or socioeconomic status.

In summary, cardiovascular diseases are undergoing a therapeutic revolution. Innovations in gene therapy, medical imaging, and nanotechnology offer unprecedented opportunities for patient care. While challenges persist, ongoing innovation and research hold promise for more effective management or even cure of cardiovascular diseases. The dedication of the scientific and medical communities, bolstered by supportive public health policies and equitable access to care, is essential for translating these hopes into reality and fostering a healthier future for all.

CONCLUSION

It's crucial to reflect on the wealth of knowledge we've acquired and the transformative potential it holds for our lives. Armed with evidence-based strategies and practical advice, we stand at the forefront of proactive heart health management. From understanding the importance of a heart-healthy diet to embracing regular physical activity and stress-reducing techniques, we've laid the foundation for long-term cardiovascular well-being.

Moving forward, let us remember that prevention is key. By adopting healthy lifestyle habits and adhering to medical recommendations, we can significantly reduce our risk of developing heart disease and its complications. Moreover, for those already facing heart-related challenges, the tools provided in this book offer hope and empowerment. Through diligent implementation of the outlined strategies, individuals can take control of their health outcomes and work toward reversing the course of heart disease.

Furthermore, let us not overlook the importance of ongoing education and collaboration with healthcare professionals. As new research emerges and medical advancements continue, staying informed and engaged ensures that we remain proactive in our approach to heart health.

Finally, this guide serves as a valuable resource, equipping readers with the knowledge and tools necessary to safeguard their cardiovascular well-being. Let us embrace these insights and look at the pathway towards a heart-healthy future filled with vitality and longevity.